Copyright © 2023 by Williams Charlotte

All rights reserved. No part of this publication may be reproduced, distributed, or transmitted in any form or by any means, including photocopying, recording, or other electronic or mechanical methods, without the prior written permission of the publisher, except in the case of brief quotation embodied in critical reviews and certain other noncommercial uses permitted by copyright law.

Contents

Introduction 5
What is Hepatitis A? 6
How is Hepatitis A transmitted? 6
What are the symptoms of Hepatitis A? 7
Why is prevention and management important? 7
Hepatitis A Prevention 8
Vaccination: Who Should Get It and How Effective Is It? ... 8
Proper Hand Hygiene and Sanitation 8
Safe Food Handling Practices 9
Travel Tips for Hepatitis A Prevention 9
Nutritional Considerations for Hepatitis A 10
The Importance of Proper Nutrition 10
Key Nutrients for Hepatitis A 11
Tips for Maintaining Proper Nutrition 12
Hepatitis A-Friendly Recipes 13
   Carrot and Radish Slaw with Mint-Turmeric 14
   Meatloaf 15
   Moroccan-Inspired Breakfast Skillet 17
   Coleslaw stir fry 19
   Shrimp Scampi 20

Coconut Crusted Cod with Mango Salsa ... 21

Vegan Pesto Pizza Recipe ... 23

Mediterranean chicken salad ... 25

SPECIAL AUTOIMMUNE RECIPE FOR BREAKFAST ... 27

Sweet Potato Avocado Toast ... 27

Cauliflower Maple Raisin Overnight N'Oatmeal ... 28

Pumpkin bars ... 29

Mediterranean Cauliflower Couscous Salad ... 30

Parsnip risotto ... 33

Honey lime shrimp bowl ... 34

Tropical chicken salad ... 36

Butternut Soup ... 39

1-2-3 Hash ... 40

Autoimmune Breakfast Sausages ... 41

Cranberry-Braised Short Ribs ... 42

One pan taco skillet ... 43

Chicken salad with honey lemon dressing ... 45

BBQ sauce ... 46

Shrimp Scampi ... 48

Ribboned asparagus and fennel salad ... 49

Night shade curry ... 50

Blueberry muffins 52

Paleo Pesto 54

Carrot and sweet potato chili 55

Green curry 56

Radish Slaw with Mint-Turmeric Pesto 58

Strawberry and cream tart 59

Green soup 62

Fermented pickles 64

Salmon Stew with Rutabaga, Leeks, and Dill 68

Guacamole recipe 70

Pumpkin soup 71

Shredded chicken 73

Roasted butternut squash 78

Meal Planning and Preparation Tips for Hepatitis A 79

Conclusion 81

Introduction

Hepatitis A is a viral infection that affects the liver. It is caused by the Hepatitis A virus, which is primarily spread through contaminated food and water or close personal contact with an infected person. Hepatitis A can cause a range of symptoms, including fever, nausea, vomiting, abdominal pain, fatigue, and jaundice. While most people recover fully from Hepatitis A, some individuals may experience severe symptoms and complications, particularly those with pre-existing liver disease.

The purpose of this book is to provide a comprehensive guide to Hepatitis A, including prevention and management strategies, nutritional considerations, lifestyle management tips, and information on Hepatitis A in special populations. By understanding the causes, symptoms, and management of Hepatitis A, individuals can take proactive steps to protect their health and well-being.

In this chapter, we will provide an overview of Hepatitis A, including how it is transmitted, its symptoms and complications, and the importance of prevention and management.

What is Hepatitis A?

Hepatitis A is a viral infection that affects the liver. It is one of several types of viral hepatitis, including Hepatitis B and C. While all forms of viral hepatitis can cause liver damage, each virus is transmitted differently and may require different treatment strategies.

How is Hepatitis A transmitted?

Hepatitis A is primarily spread through the fecal-oral route. This means that the virus is passed from an infected person to an uninfected person through contact with infected fecal matter. This can occur through contaminated food and water or close personal contact with an infected person. Hepatitis A can also be spread through sexual contact or the sharing of needles with an infected person.

What are the symptoms of Hepatitis A?

Symptoms of Hepatitis A can range from mild to severe and may include fever, nausea, vomiting, abdominal pain, fatigue, and jaundice (yellowing of the skin and eyes). While most people recover fully from Hepatitis A, some individuals may experience severe symptoms and complications, particularly those with pre-existing liver disease.

Why is prevention and management important?

Prevention and management are critical for protecting individuals from Hepatitis A and minimizing the risk of severe complications. Prevention strategies include vaccination, proper hand hygiene and sanitation, safe food handling practices, and travel precautions. Management strategies include symptom management, nutritional support, and lifestyle management, as well as medical treatment when necessary

Hepatitis A Prevention

Preventing Hepatitis A is critical for maintaining overall health and well-being. While there is no specific treatment for Hepatitis A, the virus can be prevented through a range of strategies, including vaccination, proper hand hygiene and sanitation, safe food handling practices, and travel precautions.

Vaccination: Who Should Get It and How Effective Is It?

The Hepatitis A vaccine is highly effective at preventing the virus. The vaccine is recommended for all children at the age of one year, individuals who are at increased risk of Hepatitis A infection, and travelers to areas with high rates of Hepatitis A. The vaccine is given in two doses, six months apart, and provides long-term protection against the virus.

Proper Hand Hygiene and Sanitation

Proper hand hygiene is essential for preventing the spread of Hepatitis A. Individuals should wash their hands thoroughly with soap and water for at least 20 seconds after using the bathroom, changing diapers, and before preparing or consuming food. It is also important to use clean and safe drinking water, and to avoid sharing personal items like towels or toothbrushes.

Safe Food Handling Practices

Hepatitis A can be transmitted through contaminated food, so it is important to practice safe food handling practices. This includes washing fruits and vegetables thoroughly, cooking meat and poultry to the appropriate temperature, and avoiding raw or undercooked shellfish. Individuals should also avoid eating food from street vendors and other locations that may not have adequate food safety measures in place.

Travel Tips for Hepatitis A Prevention

Travelers to areas with high rates of Hepatitis A should take extra precautions to prevent infection. This includes receiving the Hepatitis A vaccine before travel, avoiding street food and raw or undercooked food, and only drinking bottled water or boiled water. It is also important to practice good hand hygiene and avoid close personal contact with individuals who may be infected.

Nutritional Considerations for Hepatitis A

Maintaining a healthy and balanced diet is important for overall health and well-being, and it is particularly important for individuals with Hepatitis A. Proper nutrition can help support liver function, manage symptoms, and promote overall recovery. In this chapter, we will explore the nutritional considerations for individuals with Hepatitis A.

The Importance of Proper Nutrition

Hepatitis A can cause a range of symptoms, including nausea, vomiting, abdominal pain, and loss of appetite. These symptoms can make it challenging to maintain proper nutrition, which is essential for supporting liver function and overall health. Proper nutrition can also help manage symptoms, support immune function, and promote overall recovery.

Key Nutrients for Hepatitis A

There are several key nutrients that are particularly important for individuals with Hepatitis A, including:

Protein: Protein is essential for maintaining liver function and repairing damaged tissues. Good sources of protein include lean meats, poultry, fish, beans, and nuts.

Carbohydrates: Carbohydrates provide energy and can help manage symptoms like fatigue. Good sources of carbohydrates include fruits, vegetables, whole grains, and starchy vegetables like potatoes and sweet potatoes.

Healthy Fats: Healthy fats, such as those found in nuts, seeds, and fatty fish, can help reduce inflammation and support liver function.

Vitamins and Minerals: Vitamins and minerals, such as vitamin A, vitamin C, vitamin E, and zinc, are essential for immune function and overall health. Good sources of these nutrients include fruits, vegetables, whole grains, and lean meats.

Tips for Maintaining Proper Nutrition

Maintaining proper nutrition can be challenging for individuals with Hepatitis A, particularly during periods of illness or decreased appetite. Here are some tips for maintaining proper nutrition:

Eat small, frequent meals throughout the day to manage symptoms and prevent nausea.

Focus on nutrient-dense foods, such as fruits, vegetables, lean proteins, and whole grains.

Stay hydrated by drinking plenty of fluids, such as water, herbal tea, and low-sugar sports drinks.

Avoid alcohol and other substances that can further damage the liver.

Hepatitis A-Friendly Recipes

Maintaining proper nutrition is important for individuals with Hepatitis A, but it can be challenging to find recipes that are both flavorful and gentle on the liver. In this chapter, we will explore a range of Hepatitis A-friendly recipes that are packed with nutrients and flavor.

Carrot and Radish Slaw with Mint-Turmeric

INGREDIENTS

6 medium carrots (about ¾ pound), peeled

5 large radishes

1-inch piece peeled ginger

1 half ripe avocado

⅔ cup tightly packed mint leaves

⅓ cup tightly packed cilantro leaves

1 large cove garlic, chopped

1 tablespoon lemon juice

1 teaspoon ground turmeric

½ teaspoon salt

3 tablespoons olive oil

1 tablespoon water

Fresh lemon for serving

INSTRUCTIONS

Using the S-blade of your food processor, shred the carrots, radishes and ginger. If you do not have a food processor, you can grate the vegetables. Transfer to a serving bowl.

Clean out the food processor. Add the avocado, herbs, garlic, lemon, turmeric and salt to the bowl of the food processor. Combine until the herbs are finely chopped.

With the food processor running, slowly drizzle in the olive oil and water to emulsify the pesto.

Toss the pesto with the shredded vegetables in the serving bowl. Serve with a squeeze of fresh lemon juice, if desired.

Meatloaf
INGREDIENTS

1 tablespoon coconut oil

1 cup cauliflower, processed into "rice" with a food processor

1 zucchini, peeled and grated

1 carrot, peeled and grated

½ onion, minced

4 cloves garlic, minced

½ cup parsley, chopped

2 teaspoons sea salt

2 tablespoons fresh thyme and/or marjoram

2 egg yolks (omit if on the elimination diet)

2 lbs ground beef, lamb, or pork mixture (I used beef and lamb), room temperature

3-4 slices pastured bacon

INSTRUCTIONS

Preheat your oven to 350 degrees. In a skillet, heat the coconut oil and saute the onion, zucchini, carrot and cauliflower rice for about 5 minutes, adding the garlic at the very end. Let cool.

In a large bowl mix the egg yolks with the herbs and spices including the fresh parsley. Add the meat and vegetables to the bowl. Mix gently with your hands until just incorporated.

Transfer the mixture to a 9 x 5 loaf pan, making sure to spread it evenly into the corners. Lay the bacon strips across the top, tucking them in to the ends if they are too long. Cook for 45-50 minutes, or until the internal temperature reaches 155 degrees. Remove from oven and carefully pour off liquid, reserving it to cook veggies in later.

Put the loaf back in the oven for 10 minutes under the broiler to crisp up the bacon. Let sit for 10 minutes before slicing.

Moroccan-Inspired Breakfast Skillet

Ingredients

1 lb pastured ground pork

2 tablespoons solid cooking fat (coconut oil or lard work well here)

1 medium sweet potato, diced (about 2 cups)

1 small bunch chard, stems removed, separated, and both stems and leaves chopped

3 cloves garlic, minced

1 teaspoon ground turmeric

½ teaspoon sea salt

⅛ teaspoon cinnamon

1 teaspoon apple cider vinegar

½ cup raisins

Instructions

Place the ground pork in the bottom of a cold heavy-bottomed pan, and break up slightly with a utensil. Turn on medium-high heat, and cook, stirring, until the meat is browned and has absorbed all of the fat (don't drain it off!). Turn off the heat, transfer to a large bowl and set aside.

Place the same pan back on the stove, add the solid cooking fat, and turn the heat to medium-high. When the fat has melted and the pan is hot, add the sweet potatoes and cook, stirring, for five minutes. Add the chard stems and cook for three more minutes.

Add the garlic, turmeric, sea salt, and cinnamon, and stir to combine. Cook for a few more minutes, until the sweet potatoes are just soft.

Add the chard leaves, apple cider vinegar, and raisins to the pan. Continue cooking until chard has wilted, about a minute or two. Turn off the heat, salt to taste, and serve warm!

Coleslaw stir fry

INGREDIENTS

1 tbsp coconut oil

3 cloves garlic

1 onion

5-6 Rashes Bacon, Chopped 3cm pieces

160 g red cabbage, Chopped 2-3cm

160 g green cabbage, Chopped 2-3cm

1 carrot, Chopped 2cm Pieces

Instructions

Add everything to the bowl and Chop 3 Seconds, Speed 5You may need your spatula to assist

Scrape the sides down

Repeat step 1, Chop 3 Seconds, Speed 5You may need your spatula to assist

Pour into your Wok or Frying pan on a medium heat

Stir until coleslaw is softened and slightly translucent, approximately 10 minutes

Place into thermoserver or serve immediately

Shrimp Scampi

INGREDIENTS

⅓ cup extra virgin olive oil

3 garlic cloves, minced

1 lb shrimp, peeled

⅓ cup dry white wine or bone broth

1 tbsp lemon juice

¼ cup parsley, chopped

INSTRUCTIONS

Cook the garlic in the olive oil over medium heat, stirring occasionally, for five minutes.

Raise the heat to medium-high and add the shrimp. Cook, stirring, another five minutes, until the shrimp is done.

Add the wine and butter and cook another minute, then add the lemon juice and stir well.

Garnish with the parsley to serve.

Coconut Crusted Cod with Mango Salsa
INGREDIENTS

Salsa Ingredients

1 large mango, peeled and diced

1 avocado, cubed

½ small red onion, diced

1 cucumber, diced

1 bunch cilantro, chopped

2 cloves garlic, minced

½ teaspoon sea salt

1 tablespoon olive oil

1 lime, juiced

Fish Ingredients

24 ounces cod fillets, cut into 2 inch thick strips

1 ½ cups coconut flour

1 ½ teaspoons ginger powder

¼ teaspoon sea salt

2 cups coconut milk

1 cup finely shredded coconut

2 tablespoons coconut oil

Mango salsa (see above)

INSTRUCTIONS

First prepare the mango salsa and set aside.

Wash, dry, and debone the cod fillets.

Combine the coconut flour, ginger powder and salt on a plate or shallow bowl. Place the coconut milk in another shallow bowl, as well as the shredded coconut. Dip the cod strips into the coconut milk, then the coconut flour mixture, back into the coconut milk, and finally into the shredded coconut, paying special attention to creating a thick breading.

Heat the coconut oil in a large skillet on medium-high heat. When it is hot, cook the cod strips for five minutes a side depending on thickness of the fish, or until the top and bottom are nice and browned and the fish is cooked throughout. Once the cod strips are in the pan, try not to fuss with them too much – because there is no egg in the breading, they are a little delicate.

Serve with mango salsa.

Vegan Pesto Pizza Recipe
INGREDIENTS

2 ½ cups Gluten Free All Purpose Flour

¼ cup Ground Flaxseed

1 ½ tbs Psyllium Husk Powder

1 tsp Baking Powder

1 tsp Sea Salt

½ tsp Instant Yeast

1 ½ cups Warm Water

½ cup Extra Virgin Olive Oil (plus more for greasing)

½ cup Dairy Free Pesto

Toppings of choice

INSTRUCTIONS

In a mixing bowl, combine flaxseed, psyllium husk, baking powder, salt, and yeast.

Add the warm water and oil. Mix with a fork, then knead with your hands and form a ball. The dough should be a bit sticky, but hold it's shape. If too wet, add more psyllium husk. If too dry, add water. Cover with a damp towel and let sit at room temperature for 60 minutes.

Adjust the oven racks to the top and preheat the oven to 500 F. Place a pizza stone or baking sheet in the oven.

Grease your fingers with a bit of olive oil. Transfer the dough to a piece of aluminum foil and gently press into a thin, round layer, roughly ¼" thick. Transfer into the preheating stone or sheet and bake for 8 to 10 minutes.

Spread the pesto evenly over the pizza and top with toppings. Bake for an additional 7 to 9 minutes. Let cool slightly and enjoy!

NOTES

You can refrigerate this pizza for up to 7 days in an airtight container or freeze it for up to 3 months. We all know pizza is amazing even when reheated!

Mediterranean chicken salad

INGREDIENTS

For the salad:

2 cups pre-cooked chicken

½ cup shredded raw zucchini

¼ cup chopped Kalamata olives

2 tablespoons chopped fresh basil

3 cloves garlic, minced

Zest of one lemon

Salad greens or 2 hollowed out cucumbers

For the dressing:

2 tablespoons fresh-squeezed lemon juice

2 tablespoons extra virgin olive oil

1 tablespoons coconut milk (optional)

½ teaspoon sea salt, or to taste

INSTRUCTIONS

In a large bowl, mix together chicken, zucchini, olives, basil, garlic, and lemon zest.

In a smaller bowl, whisk dressing ingredients: lemon juice, olive oil, coconut milk (if using), and salt.

Add dressing to the chicken mixture, and stir well to combine.

To serve, place two cucumber quarters on each plate, or greens drizzled with a little olive oil. Top with chicken salad.

SPECIAL AUTOIMMUNE RECIPE FOR BREAKFAST

Sweet Potato Avocado Toast

Ingredients

1 large sweet potato, skin-on, sliced into ¼"-thick toast shapes

2 tsp olive oil

1 medium avocado, thinly sliced

Lemon juice, to drizzle

Sea salt, to taste

Instructions

Place your oven's rack at the slot second to the top. Preheat your oven's broiler to 450 or set it to HIGH.

Place the sweet potato slices on a medium sheet pan. Drizzle the olive oil over the top, then use a pastry brush or your hands to coat both sides of the sweet potato slices.

Arrange the slices in a single layer, then broil for 5 minutes on each side or until golden brown and al dente.

Serve sweet potato toasts topped with avocado slices, lemon juice, and sea salt.

Recipe Notes

For extra protein, add cooked and crumbled AIP compliant bacon on top when serving.

Cauliflower Maple Raisin Overnight N'Oatmeal
Ingredients

1 lb fresh or frozen riced cauliflower, steamed, sauteed, or microwaved until tender

2 cups coconut milk or tigernut milk

2 Tbsp coconut flour (or ¼ cup tigernut flour)

¼ cup collagen powder

¼ cup unsulphured, unsweetened raisins

1 tsp ground cinnamon

⅛ tsp sea salt

1-2 Tbsp pure maple syrup (optional)

Instructions

Add all ingredients to a medium mixing bowl. Stir well to combine, then taste and adjust seasonings if desired.

Divide mixture evenly between 4 mason jars. Cover then refrigerate overnight or for at least 4 hours. N'oatmeal is ready when the mixture has thickened and the raisins are soft.

Recipe Notes

Top with toasted sliced tigernuts just before serving for an extra crunch!

Pumpkin bars

Ingredients

½ cup coconut manna or butter

½ cup coconut oil

¼ cup heaping coconut flour

1 ½ cups winter squash (butternut, pumpkin, acorn)

1 pinch salt

2 teaspoons cinnamon

1 teaspoon ground ginger

1/3 cup maple syrup

Instructions

On the stove, gently melt coconut oil and manna until creamy and lump free

In food processor, add squash, spices, coconut flour, salt and maple syrup. Pour melted coconut oil and manna on top and blend for 30 seconds being sure all the big pieces of squash are blended

Line a square 8x8 brownie pan with parchment paper. Scoop the bar filling into the pan and use a spatula to smooth it out. Bake for 25 min at 350 degrees. Remove from oven, let cool, cover and put in fridge until completely chilled; about 3 hours

Mediterranean Cauliflower Couscous Salad

INGREDIENTS

1 tbsp olive oil

3½ cups uncooked riced cauliflower

¼ tsp sea salt

¾ cup peeled, seeded, and diced cucumber

⅔ cup finely chopped parsley, loosely packed

½ cup dried cranberries

⅓ cup diced dried Turkish figs

⅓ cup diced red onion

4 green onions, sliced crosswise

1 tbsp minced fresh dill

Vinaigrette:

3 tbsp olive oil

1 tbsp + ½ tsp lemon juice

1 tbsp apple cider vinegar

½ tsp grated orange zest

½ tsp sea salt

¼ tsp garlic powder

¼ tsp dried dill

INSTRUCTIONS

Heat olive oil in a large stainless steel pan over medium heat.

Add riced cauliflower to the pan and season with sea salt. Saute for 5 minutes, tossing only every 2 minutes to prevent sticking, until lightly browned and tender. Ensure you do not overcook the rice or it will be mushy.

Set the cooked cauliflower rice aside to cool completely. You may do this by leaving it at room temperature for 30 minutes or by scooping onto a plate and placing in the refrigerator until cooled.

Meanwhile, combine the remaining salad ingredients in a serving bowl. Toss in the cooled and cooked riced cauliflower.

Make the vinaigrette by whisking all of its ingredients together in a small bowl. Toss gently with the salad until evenly incorporated.

Parsnip risotto

INGREDIENTS

1½ pounds parsnips, riced (see note below)

1 tablespoon solid cooking fat

½ yellow onion, minced

1 cup finely chopped mushrooms

3 cloves minced garlic

2 tablespoons minced fresh sage

½ teaspoon sea salt

1 teaspoon apple cider vinegar

¾ cup bone broth

INSTRUCTIONS

Heat the cooking fat in a large skillet or heavy-bottomed pot on medium heat. When the fat has melted and the pan is hot, add the onions and mushrooms. Cook, stirring, until the onions are translucent, about 5 minutes. Add the garlic, sage, and sea salt, and cook for another 2 minutes, just until fragrant.

Add the apple cider vinegar and scrape up any bits that have stuck to the bottom of the pan. Add the processed parsnips and bone broth to the pan, stirring to incorporate. Cook for 5 to 7 minutes, uncovered, on medium heat, stirring occasionally, until the liquid has been absorbed and the parsnips are fully cooked

Honey lime shrimp bowl

INGREDIENTS

⅓ cup honey

¼ cup coconut aminos

2 garlic cloves, crushed

1 teaspoon minced fresh ginger

1 lb medium uncooked shrimp, peeled and deveined

Olive oil for sautéing

Salad greens

Cooked cauliflower rice

Veggies/fruit of choice

Sea salt as desired for seasoning shrimp

Optional: chopped cilantro or green onion for garnish

INSTRUCTIONS

Place shrimp, garlic and sea salt in a container to marinate 30 minutes to an hour and set aside.

Plate your salad greens, cauliflower rice and veggies and/or fruit of choice.

Set aside.

Next, combine honey, coconut aminos, and ginger. Whisk to combine.

Heat olive oil in a pan over medium high heat.

Add marinated shrimp to pan and cook for 1 to 2 minutes per side until just opaque before adding your sauce.

Add lime juice and zest just before finishing.

Add shrimp to your bowl or dish and Enjoy!

Tropical chicken salad

Ingredients

2 skinless chicken breasts

1 small head red leaf lettuce (or similar), washed and torn

1 cup ripe mango, diced

¼ small red onion, thinly sliced

½ ripe avocado

1 lime, juiced

3 Tbsp extra virgin olive oil

1 bunch of fresh cilantro

½ cup green plantain chips (homemade or bought)

¼ cup shredded unsweetened coconut

Instructions:

Clean chicken breasts and place at the bottom of a pot. Season with kosher salt and cover with water by 2 inches. Bring to a boil, then reduce heat to low and cover. Cook for approx. 8 minutes (the internal temp. should at least be 165f degrees).

When the chicken is done, add it to a plate and with two forks, pull at the chicken breasts to shred. Set aside.

Make the salad dressing by combining: lime juice, oil, and finely chopped cilantro to a food processor or just shaking it in a mason jar.

Assemble the salad by adding torn lettuce to bowls and dress with the salad dressing.

Top with diced mango, sliced red onion, avocado slices, plantain chips, shredded coconut, and chicken. Serve!

Carrot and Sweet Potato "Chili"

INGREDIENTS

2 tablespoons solid cooking fat

1 onion, chopped

8 cloves garlic, minced

1 tablespoon fresh thyme

2 cups carrots, cut into large chunks

4 cups sweet potatoes, cut into large chunks

4 cups bone broth

1 teaspoon sea salt

2 pounds grass-fed ground beef

1-2 avocados

Cilantro for garnish

INSTRUCTIONS

Heat your cooking fat in the bottom of a heavy-bottomed pot. Add the onion and cook for a few minutes, until translucent. Add the garlic and thyme and cook for another couple of minutes, stirring.

Add the carrots and sweet potatoes and cook for 5 minutes, or until gently browned. Add the bone broth and sea salt and bring to a boil, cover and then simmer for 20 minutes, until the vegetables are soft.

Meanwhile, cook the ground beef in a skillet until thoroughly cooked throughout and browned. Set aside.

When the vegetables are finished, add the ground beef and stir to combine. Continue cooking for another 15 minutes covered at a simmer. Serve each bowl garnished with avocado slices and fresh parsley.

Butternut Soup

Ingredients

12 oz fresh or frozen chopped butternut squash

1 cup frozen chopped onions

1 cup coconut milk or tigernut milk

2 cups AIP compliant bone broth (or more, depending on how thick you like your soup)

AIP all purpose seasoning, like Paleo Powder, to taste

Instructions

Add all ingredients to a medium soup pot over medium high heat. Cover then bring to a low boil.

Remove cover then turn down the heat to medium until it simmers moderately. Cook for 5 minutes or until squash is tender.

Turn off the heat, then carefully use an immersion blender or blend in batches in your high-speed blender until very smooth and velvety.

1-2-3 Hash

Prep Time 5 minutes

Cook Time 10 minutes

Servings 4 people

Ingredients

1 Tbsp lard or duck fat

1 lb ground pork

1 lb bag of coleslaw mix (shredded cabbage and carrots, discard any dressing)

Seasonings of choice (see notes)

Instructions

Add fat to a large skillet over medium heat. When hot, add ground pork.

Crumble the pork and cook for 5 minutes or until almost cooked through.

Stir in the coleslaw mix and your preferred seasonings, then cook for 5 minutes more or until pork is cooked through fully and the colelway mix is tender-crisp.

Autoimmune Breakfast Sausages

Tools for this recipe

Large bowl

Ingredients

Ground pork

Chopped dried chives

Dried mustard

Dried garlic powder or ½ clove of garlic, finely diced

Dried onion powder or ¼ onion, finely diced

Sea salt

Autoimmune Breakfast Sausages Instructions

Mix and mold into mini patties. Cook on medium. Makes 8 mini patties.

*I make bigger batches and freeze the sausages for a quick breakfast option.

Cranberry-Braised Short Ribs

Ingredients

1 tablespoon coconut oil

4 pounds short ribs

1/8 teaspoon sea salt

1 ½ cups chicken broth

1 cup cranberry juice

1 cup cranberries

2 tablespoons apple cider vinegar

1 whole bay leaf

2 tablespoons parsley

Equipment

Dutch oven

Instructions

Preheat the oven to 300F.

Heat the fat in a heavy-bottomed pot and sear the meat on all sides. Turn off the heat and salt to taste.

Add the remaining ingredients. Add a little bit more broth if the liquid doesn't reach 1/3 of the way up the meat.

Braise, covered, 2-3 hours in the oven. It is ready when the meat is falling off the bone.

Serve garnished with fresh parsley.

One pan taco skillet
INGREDIENTS

1 lb ground beef

1 onion, diced

2 cup cauliflower rice (pre-riced or using a food processor)

1 cup zucchini, diced

1 cup kale, thinly sliced

1 tsp sea salt

½ tsp black pepper

2 tsp oregano

2 tsp garlic powder

2 tsp cumin (sub ¼ tsp turmeric)

2 tsp chili powder

Juice of one lime

Toppings:

Dairy-free sour cream

2 tbsp green onion, chopped

2 tbsp cilantro, chopped

1 avocado, diced

¼ cup black olives, sliced

½ cup grape tomatoes, sliced (omit for AIP)

1 lime, quartered

INSTRUCTIONS

Using a large skillet, brown the ground beef over medium heat. Set aside and reserve the fat in the pan.

Saute the onion in skillet for 4-5 minutes or until translucent.

Add in the cauliflower rice and zucchini and saute until the cauliflower rice is lightly browned and the zucchini is softened.

Stir in the greens and the seasonings and saute until the greens are wilted.

Add the beef back in and cook for 2-3 minutes to combine the flavors.

Remove the heat and add the toppings. Season further to taste and serve!

Chicken salad with honey lemon dressing
INGREDIENTS

For the salad:

1 chicken breast (approx. 200 g), cooked and diced

2 strawberries or other berries or other fruits, sliced

2–3 oz (75 g) salad leaves (I like arugula)

For the dressing:

2 Tablespoons olive oil

½ teaspoon raw honey

1 teaspoon fresh lemon juice

INSTRUCTIONS

Mix all the dressing ingredients together.

Toss salad together with dressing.

BBQ sauce
Ingredients

1 Tbsp Lemon Juice, fresh squeezed + 1 tsp for other step

1 Tbsp Apple Cider Vinegar, (or red wine vinegar)

¼ cup Maple Syrup, Pure

1 Tbsp Bacon Grease

1 tsp Ginger, ground, dried, powder

1 cup Carrots, diced

1 cup Onion, diced

1 cup Strawberries, fresh, chopped

½ tsp Salt, (smoked salt)

Instructions

In a saucepan, add maple syrup, lemon juice, vinegar, ginger, onions, carrots, strawberries and bacon fat. Bring to boil, stir and lower to a simmer. Add smoked salt, stir until it has dissolved and taste the mixture for salt. You may need to add more. The amount of smoked salt you will add will be very organic and intuitive; add more if you like a lot of smoke flavor. I added three small pinches of my smoked salt.

Simmer on low for about 20 minutes or until the onions and carrots are tender.

Transfer to blender and (using a towel to cover the top of the blender lid so you don't burn yourself in case any flows over) blend on high until completely smooth, scraping down sides once or twice, about 2 minutes. Pour back into saucepan and bring to low simmer and cook for about 10 min. more. Will keep in fridge for up to 5 days. Freeze if you don't think you will use it all.

Shrimp Scampi

INGREDIENTS

⅓ cup extra virgin olive oil

3 garlic cloves, minced

1 lb shrimp, peeled

⅓ cup dry white wine or bone broth

1 tbsp lemon juice

¼ cup parsley, chopped

INSTRUCTIONS

Cook the garlic in the olive oil over medium heat, stirring occasionally, for five minutes.

Raise the heat to medium-high and add the shrimp. Cook, stirring, another five minutes, until the shrimp is done.

Add the wine and butter and cook another minute, then add the lemon juice and stir well.

Garnish with the parsley to serve

Ribboned asparagus and fennel salad

INGREDIENTS

1-2 pounds asparagus, white ends trimmed

1 large fennel bulb

¼ cup extra-virgin olive oil

1 lemon, juiced

¼ teaspoon lemon zest (here is the zester I use)

¼ teaspoon sea salt

INSTRUCTIONS

Take the asparagus and use a vegetable peeler to create long "ribbons" and place them in a bowl. I find it easiest to start towards the spear end, and then come back and do the bottoms. You will end up with a little "core" at the end; you can either slice this thin with a knife and add to the salad or discard.

Use a mandoline slicer on the thinnest setting to slice the fennel bulb. Add it to the bowl with the asparagus.

Add the olive oil, lemon juice, zest, and sea salt to the asparagus and fennel. Toss to combine.

Night shade curry

Ingredients

1 (15-ounce) can full-fat coconut milk, see note*

2 Tbsp minced ginger

3 cloves garlic, minced, optional**

2 large carrots, peeled and sliced

1 large crown broccoli, chopped into florets**

1 yellow squash, chopped

1 large boneless skinless chicken breast

2 Tbsp coconut aminos

1 tsp ground turmeric

½ tsp ground cinnamon

½ tsp sea salt, to taste

1 lime, cut into wedges

½ cup fresh basil, chopped for serving

Instructions

Pour ¼ cup of the coconut milk into a large skillet and heat to medium. Add the ginger and garlic, and cook until fragrant, about 2 to 3 minutes.

Add the carrots and broccoli and cover. Cook, stirring occasionally, until veggies have softened but are still al dente, about 3 minutes.

Heat a small amount of coconut oil or avocado oil in a separate skillet over medium heat. Add the chopped chicken. Brown the chicken, stirring occasionally, until a great deal of liquid comes out, about 5 minutes. You don't need to cook the chicken all the way through – you're simply cooking out the liquid. Strain the liquid from the chicken, then add the chicken to the skillet with the vegetables.

Add the remaining ingredients (including the rest of the coconut milk) except for the lime wedges and basil to the skillet with the vegetables and chicken. Stir well and bring to a full boil, then reduce the heat to a simmer and cover. Cook 15 minutes, then uncover and continue cooking another 8 to 10 minutes, until curry has thickened and chicken is cooked through.

Taste curry for flavor and add sea salt to taste. Serve with choice of cauliflower rice or other riced vegetables or regular rice. Garnish with lime wedges and basil.

Notes

*Be sure to get coconut milk without any added gums/emulsifiers to keep this recipe AIP

For Low-FODMAP, omit the garlic and use 1 bunch of broccolini instead of broccoli.

Blueberry muffins

Ingredients

¾ cup cassava flour Otto's brand preferred and recommended

⅓ cup lard or coconut oil, melted and cooled slightly

⅓ cup coconut milk or non-dairy milk of choice

⅓ cup coconut sugar

¼ cup collagen (see link and DISCOUNT code below in Recipe Notes)

3 Tablespoons water

3 Tablespoons coconut flour

1 Tablespoon gelatin (see link and DISCOUNT code below in Recipe Notes)

2 teaspoons apple cider vinegar

½ teaspoon baking soda , sifted

¼ teaspoon sea salt

⅓ cup blueberries frozen or fresh (but not frozen and defrosted because they'll be too wet for the batter)

Instructions

Preheat oven to 350 degrees Fahrenheit. Line muffin pan with liners or heavily grease. Set aside.

In large bowl combine dry ingredients: cassava flour, coconut sugar, collagen, coconut flour, gelatin, baking soda and sea salt.

In medium bowl combine wet ingredients: fat of choice, coconut milk, water and apple cider vinegar. Add wet ingredients to dry ingredients and stir to combine. (You may also use an electric handheld mixer.)

Fold or mix in blueberries.

Fill muffin tin with batter.

Muffin batter in pan

Bake until toothpick inserted in center comes out clean and muffins are golden brown, about 19 minutes for 6 muffins or 25 to 30 minutes for larger muffins.

Paleo Pesto

Ingredients

2 cups fresh basil

2 tablespoons fresh oregano

1/3 cup shredded unsweetened coconut

1 tablespoon fresh lemon juice

¼ cup olive oil

1 clove garlic

1 pinch salt

Instructions

In a food processor add all the ingredients and blend for 30 seconds, taking time to scrape down sides once with spatula.

Store in airtight glass container in fridge for up to 4 days

Carrot and sweet potato chili

INGREDIENTS

2 tablespoons solid cooking fat

1 onion, chopped

8 cloves garlic, minced

1 tablespoon fresh thyme

2 cups carrots, cut into large chunks

4 cups sweet potatoes, cut into large chunks

4 cups bone broth

1 teaspoon sea salt

2 pounds grass-fed ground beef

1-2 avocados

Cilantro for garnish

INSTRUCTIONS

Heat your cooking fat in the bottom of a heavy-bottomed pot. Add the onion and cook for a few minutes, until translucent. Add the garlic and thyme and cook for another couple of minutes, stirring.

Add the carrots and sweet potatoes and cook for 5 minutes, or until gently browned. Add the bone broth and sea salt and bring to a boil, cover and then simmer for 20 minutes, until the vegetables are soft.

Meanwhile, cook the ground beef in a skillet until thoroughly cooked throughout and browned. Set aside.

When the vegetables are finished, add the ground beef and stir to combine. Continue cooking for another 15 minutes covered at a simmer. Serve each bowl garnished with avocado slices and fresh parsley.

Green curry

INGREDIENTS

2 tbsp coconut oil

½ large yellow onion, chopped

3-4 stalks lemongrass, exterior removed and chopped (about ¼ cup)

1½ tbsp minced fresh ginger

1½ tbsp minced fresh turmeric

3 cloves garlic, minced

1 bunch cilantro, ⅔ cup including stem ends roughly chopped and the tops reserved

1 can coconut milk (either thickener-free or homemade)

½ tsp sea salt

2 limes, juiced

INSTRUCTIONS

Heat the coconut oil in the bottom of a skillet or heavy-bottomed pot on medium-high heat. When the fat has melted and the pan is hot, add the onions and sauté for 7 minutes, until translucent, stirring occasionally.

Add the lemongrass, ginger, turmeric, garlic, and cilantro (2/3 of the bunch including the stem ends) to the pan and cook for 3 minutes, stirring.

Add the coconut milk and sea salt, turn down to a simmer, and cook for 10 minutes.

Turn off the heat and set aside for a few minutes to cool.

When the mixture is cool enough to handle, add the lime juice and transfer to a blender. Blend on high until well incorporated, for 60 seconds or so.

Add salt to taste and serve with protein of your choice garnished with remaining cilantro leaves

Radish Slaw with Mint-Turmeric Pesto

INGREDIENTS

6 medium carrots (about ¾ pound), peeled

5 large radishes

1-inch piece peeled ginger

1 half ripe avocado

⅔ cup tightly packed mint leaves

⅓ cup tightly packed cilantro leaves

1 large cove garlic, chopped

1 tablespoon lemon juice

1 teaspoon ground turmeric

½ teaspoon salt

3 tablespoons olive oil

1 tablespoon water

Fresh lemon for serving

INSTRUCTIONS

Using the S-blade of your food processor, shred the carrots, radishes and ginger. If you do not have a food processor, you can grate the vegetables. Transfer to a serving bowl.

Clean out the food processor. Add the avocado, herbs, garlic, lemon, turmeric and salt to the bowl of the food processor. Combine until the herbs are finely chopped.

With the food processor running, slowly drizzle in the olive oil and water to emulsify the pesto.

Toss the pesto with the shredded vegetables in the serving bowl. Serve with a squeeze of fresh lemon juice, if desired.

Strawberry and cream tart
Ingredients

Crust:

1 1/3 cup organic shredded coconut

1 cup of dates

Cream Filling:

1 ¾ cups coconut milk

1/3 cup dates

2 tbsp. grass-fed gelatin

¼ cup arrowroot flour

1 ½ tbsp. organic coconut oil

Strawberry Swirl:

2 cups organic strawberries

2 tbsp. organic coconut oil

2 tbsp. grass-fed gelatin

¼ cup coconut milk

Instructions

Preheat over to 325.

Before you start, your dates need to be completely softened. You can do this either by soaking them overnight or steaming them over boiling water for about 7 minutes.

For the crust:

In a high-speed blender or food processor, cream your shredded coconut. To do this, process the coconut until it has formed a thick, oily paste.

Once your coconut is creamed, add 1 cup of softened dates. Process until you had a dark, thick, dough. It will appear oily, and slightly crumbly. Your crust mixture will become more cohesive once you begin pressing the mixture into your pan.

Press your mixture down evenly into an 8" spring-form pan. Bake for 20-25 minutes, or until the edges begin to turn brown. Once your crust Is done, set it aside and allow it to cool while you prepare the filling.

For the cream filling:

Blend coconut milk (you can make your own), dates, gelatin, arrowroot flour, and coconut oil. Blend until well combined. Pour this mixture into your springform pan, on top of your crust.

For strawberry swirl:

Blend strawberries (you may use either fresh, or frozen strawberries that have been steamed and completely thawed), coconut oil, gelatin, and coconut milk. Blend completely.

Allow 5-7 minutes before pouring into cream mixture. This allows the cream to "set" so that you get the swirly design on top.

Slowly pour the strawberry mixture into the cream. I poured mine in a sporadic design and used a butter knife to create a design.

Refrigerate, and allow to set for at least 2 hours before cutting

Green soup
INGREDIENTS

2 tbsp solid cooking fat (coconut oil works great here)

1 large onion, chopped

3 cloves garlic, minced

2-in piece ginger, peeled and minced

3 cups bone broth

1 medium white sweet potato, cubed (about 3 cups)

2 small/1 large head of broccoli, chopped (about 1 cup)

1 bunch kale, chopped

1 lemon, ½ zested and juice reserved

½ tsp sea salt

1 bunch cilantro

Avocado for garnish

INSTRUCTIONS

Place the fat in the bottom of a heavy-bottomed pot on medium heat. When the fat has melted and the pan is hot, add the onions, and cook, stirring, for 5-7 minutes, or until lightly browned and translucent. Add the garlic and ginger, and cook for another minute, or until fragrant.

Add the bone broth, sweet potato, and broccoli to the pot and bring to a boil. Turn down to a simmer, cover, and cook for 10-15 minutes, or until the vegetables are tender.

Turn off the heat, add the kale, half of the bunch of cilantro, lemon zest and juice, and sea salt.

Let cool for a few minutes, and blend with a high-powered blender or immersion blender until smooth.

Serve warm garnished with avocado and cilantro.

NOTES

Note: Keeps for a week in the refrigerator and freezes well.

Fermented pickles

You will need: a medium saucepan; wooden stirring spoon; measuring cups & spoons, half gallon jar or two quart jars; airlocks/fermenting lids & weights (recommended); mortar & pestle to grind seasonings (recommended); a widemouth canning funnel is also a great tool I recommend

Ingredients:

6-10 firm pickling cucumbers or enough to pack up to the shoulder of the jar.

2.5 TBSP non-iodized, additive-free salt (e.g. pure sea salt, Morton's pickling salt, Pink Himalayan, etc.)

4 cups filtered or distilled water

4 cloves garlic, quartered (~20g)

1/8 onion thin sliced (~50-60g)

5-6 cloves, crushed (use a mortar and pestle or place in a plastic bag and use a rolling pin)

2 bay leaves (leave whole, don't crush)

Small finger of turmeric root, ~10-15g, sliced (or substitute ¼ tsp powdered)

Small finger of ginger root, ~10-15g, sliced (or substitute ¼ tsp powdered

Instructions

> In the saucepan, combine the water, salt, turmeric, cloves, and ginger, and heat on medium-high, stirring until the salt dissolves. Reduce heat and simmer for another couple minutes. (Note you will need to allow this

spiced brine to fall to room temperatures before adding it to your pickles.)

While simmering, rinse your cucumbers. Thin slice your onion and peel & quarter your garlic.

Place all the onions, garlic, and bay leaves at the bottom of the jar. (Add any herbs to the top of the jar once the cukes are in place.) Although you will likely have some floaters, we will try to keep them contained under the cucumbers as much as possible.

Add the cucumbers. Placing them firmly into place so they don't move/rise is a good approach but if it isn't possible don't stress. Try to position them so they are held in place and you can fit as many into the jar as possible. If using herbs, place them on top (these will be removed once the pickles are refrigerated, or within a week after refrigerating).

Once the brine (saltwater solution) has cooled to room temperature, slowly add it to your jar. You probably won't need to use all of it, as you want to have about 3" of space between your brine line and the rim. This water level will rise after the next step.

Once the brine was added, you may have noticed some of the spices or produce (including even the cucumbers) began to rise to the surface. You want to ensure everything is submerged under the brine. To do so, you should now add your fermenting weight. If you don't have a weight, you will likely be okay if you manage to keep all the cucumbers locked in place under the brine by packing them

At this point, everything should appear submerged, with at least a ½" airspace ("headspace") between the brine and the lid. You may now add your lid, whether that be a standard lid or an airlock lid. Sit on a shelf or your counter.

Using a fermenting weight will help ensure all produce stays below the brine. Failure to do so can result in mold growths on the exposed surfaces.

Everything is submerged and your jar is already in the process of fermenting!

For half sours, you should wait 3-5 days. For full sours, the wait is usually about a week with some extra time in the refrigerator. (Longer at room temp is a risk for mushiness.) As time passes, they will continually sour and build flavor.

Salmon Stew with Rutabaga, Leeks, and Dill

INGREDIENTS

1 tablespoon solid cooking fat

2 large leeks, ends trimmed and whites chopped into ½-inch rounds

3 cloves garlic, minced

3 cups bone broth (2 cups for the Instant Pot version)

2 cups water

2 large rutabaga, chopped into ¾-inch pieces (about 6 cups)

4 large carrots, chopped into ¾-inch pieces (about 4 cups)

4 ribs celery, chopped (about 2 cups)

3 tablespoons minced fresh dill

1 teaspoon sea salt

1 ½ pounds salmon, skinned, deboned, and cut into 1-inch chunks

½ lemon, juiced

INSTRUCTIONS

STOVETOP:

Place the fat in the bottom of a soup pot on medium heat. When the fat has melted and the pan is hot, add the leeks and cook, stirring, for about 5 minutes or until just starting to brown. Add the garlic and cook for another 30 seconds, until fragrant.

Add the broth and water to the pot, along with the rutabaga, carrots, celery, dill, and sea salt. Cover and bring to a boil; immediately turn down to a bare simmer and cook for 30 minutes, or until vegetables are fork-tender. Turn off the heat.

Gently stir in the salmon. Wait a minute or two until the pieces of salmon have turned a opaque pink and flake when probed gently; now add the lemon.

Salt to taste; serve warm.

INSTANT POT:

Follow step 1 as written above using the Saute function on your Instant Pot.

Add 2 cups of broth, the water, rutabaga, carrots, celery, dill, and sea salt to the pot. Close and lock the lid and cook on Manual – High Pressure for 7 minutes.

When the alarm goes off, use the quick-release method to release the pressure. Gently stir in the salmon. Wait a minute or two until the pieces of salmon have turned a opaque pink and flake when probed gently; now add the lemon.

Salt to taste; serve warm.

Guacamole recipe
2 large avocados

2 large garlic cloves, minced

¼ cup fresh cilantro, chopped

½ tsp onion powder

¼ tsp pepper

1 tsp sea salt or Himalayan salt

1 lime, juiced

INSTRUCTIONS

Peel the garlic then mince. Chop a handful of cilantro leaves until you fill ¼ cup. Place garlic and cilantro in a medium-size mixing bowl.

Pour salt, onion powder, pepper, and cayenne into the mixing bowl

Cut the avocados in half lengthwise and discard the pits. Use a spoon to scoop out the meat and place it in the mixing bowl.

Juice the lime by using a lime juicer or by hand.

If juicing by hand: roll the lime under the palm of your hand against the countertop or cutting board (imagine you were shaping play-dough into a ball). This will express the juice and ensure you get all the delicious lime flavor. Cut the lime in half and squeeze the juice into the bowl.

Use a fork to mash all the ingredients in the bowl together until just mixed

Serve or refrigerate for later (for up to 3-5 days)

Pumpkin soup

EQUIPMENT

Slow cooker

Blender

INGREDIENTS

2 large sweet potatoes, peeled and cubed

1 pumpkin, peeled and cubed

2 apples, cored and chopped

2 tbsp sea salt

1 tsp garlic powder

1 tsp onion powder

1 tsp turmeric powder

1 tsp ginger powder

1 tsp cinnamon powder

1 large white onion, roughly chopped

4 cups bone broth

1 Fresh sage and thyme

1 cup organic coconut milk, canned

INSTRUCTIONS

Once you've chopped the pumpkin, sweet potatoes, and apples, add them to a large bowl with the sea salt, garlic powder, onion powder, turmeric powder, ginger powder, and cinnamon powder and stir well to coat evenly.

Add the bone broth, onion, and fresh herbs to the slow cooker.

Transfer the vegetables and apples to the slow cooker and secure with the lid.

Cook on high for 6 hours. You can give the vegetables a quick stir midway through the cook. The bone broth is not meant to cover the vegetables, the steam will ensure that it cooks through.

Once your vegetables are cooked through, add your coconut milk to the pot and give it a good stir.

Transfer the mixture into the food processor and blend in batches until you reach your desired consistency. OR use a stick blender to blend into a soup

Shredded chicken
Ingredients

FOR THE DOUGH

1 ¾ cup cassava flour (more for dusting, as needed)

½ tsp fine sea salt

1 tsp cream of tartar

1 tbsp. grass fed beef gelatin

¼ + 1 tbsp cup olive oil

1 tbsp. apple cider vinegar

½ cup water (+/- as needed)

2 tbsp. olive oil (for brushing)

FOR THE CHICKEN

1 tbsp. cooking fat

1 tbsp. cooking fat

1 large onion

2 cloves garlic

lbs boneless skinless chicken thighs

1 tsp fine sea salt

1 cup compliant sauerkraut

½ cup fresh minced parsley

½ cup bone broth

2 tbsp. molasses

Instructions

Heat a large cast-iron pot or skillet on medium heat. In the meantime peel and dice the onion. Peel and mince the garlic. When the skillet has come to temperature, you can test this by drizzling water on the surface, when it dances it's ready. Add in the fat, onion and garlic. Sauté until tender.

Add in the chicken thighs and salt. Brown on all sides. Then add in the sauerkraut and the parsley. Mix well. Add in the bone broth and cover with a tight fitting lid. Lower heat to low. Cook for 20 minutes.

Remove the lid, stir in the molasses and let it simmer until the liquid is reduced by more than half. Remove from heat, use two forks to shred the chicken. Set aside.

Make the dough. You will need a large bowl, a whisk, a pastry mat or parchment paper, a rolling pin and a dough scraper or spatula.

In a large bowl mix whisk together the cassava flour, salt, cream of tartar and gelatin.

Drizzle in the olive oil and vinegar as you keep whisking until the dough gets crumbly.

Switch to a spatula. Next add in ¼ cup of warm water as you fold and mix with the spatula, add water one tablespoon at a time as needed until the dough is no longer crumbly.

Move dough to a flat surface and knead with hands until it is well combined. It should be malleable but not sticky. If it's sticky dust with flour and knead again.

Make two equal sized flat disks with the dough and wrap in plastic wrap. Set in the fridge for at least 30 minutes.

When ready to work with it again, prepare a flat surface, have the warm water at hand and more flour for dusting as needed. Unwrap one disk at a time; it will be tough and crumbly. That's fine. Let it come apart on your flat surface then add 1 to 2 tbsp. of water to the dough and knead it back to a smooth malleable consistency. Divide the dough into various equal sized balls. Each disk should make about 5 balls.

Set one ball in the center of your workspace; gently flatten with your hand. Cover with a piece of parchment paper and use a rolling pin to shape a 4-5" round, about the size of a tortilla. Use a spoon to fill with a small mound of shredded chicken. Then use spatula or dough scraper to lift the top side of the dough, gently fold it over and pinch the edges closed. You can gently roll them up a little to create a decorative boarder or use a fork to imprint on them. Scrape the empanada up and place on a baking sheet. Brush with olive oil.

Repeat this with all of the remaining dough. If some of the dough dries out as it waits its turn to be made into a lovely empanada, simply wet your fingers and massage it back to malleable texture. Alternatively, if you overdo the water on one, lightly dust it to dry up.

Once all of the empanadas are made, ensure they are spread out and not touching on the sheet pan. Place in the freezer for at least 3 hours. When they are properly frozen you can transfer them from the sheet pan to a freezer bag and store up to three months.

To heat, simply preheat your oven to 400F and place the empanada on a sheet pan. Bake for 15-20 minutes until the edges are golden.

Roasted butternut squash

INGREDIENTS

1 butternut squash, peeled, seeded and diced

2 shallots, diced

3 tablespoons coconut oil (melted)

1 teaspoon dried rosemary

1 teaspoon salt

INSTRUCTIONS

Preheat oven to 400 degrees.

Put diced squash in a large bowl and drizzle with oil. Add shallots, rosemary and salt. Stir to coat.

Spread squash in a single layer on a baking sheet.

Roast 30 minutes, stirring halfway through for even browning.

Meal Planning and Preparation Tips for Hepatitis A

Maintaining proper nutrition is important for individuals with Hepatitis A, but meal planning and preparation can be challenging during periods of illness or decreased appetite. In this chapter, we will explore a range of meal planning and preparation tips for individuals with Hepatitis A.

Plan Ahead

Meal planning is an essential tool for maintaining proper nutrition. Plan your meals and snacks ahead of time to ensure that you have nutrient-dense foods on hand when you need them. Consider prepping ingredients in advance, such as chopping vegetables or cooking grains, to make meal preparation easier and more efficient.

Focus on Nutrient-Dense Foods

Nutrient-dense foods are those that are rich in vitamins, minerals, and other essential nutrients. Focus on incorporating a variety of nutrient-dense foods into your diet, such as fruits, vegetables, whole grains, lean proteins, and healthy fats. These foods can help support liver function, manage symptoms, and promote overall recovery.

Consider Small, Frequent Meals

Eating small, frequent meals throughout the day can help manage symptoms like nausea and prevent fluctuations in blood sugar levels. Aim to eat every 2-3 hours, and focus on incorporating a mix of protein, carbohydrates, and healthy fats into each meal and snack.

Stay Hydrated

Staying hydrated is important for individuals with Hepatitis A, as dehydration can worsen symptoms and lead to further health complications. Aim to drink at least 8-10 cups of water per day, and consider incorporating low-sugar sports drinks or herbal tea for added hydration.

Avoid Alcohol and Other Substances that Can Damage the Liver

Alcohol and other substances can further damage the liver, and should be avoided by individuals with Hepatitis A. In addition, some medications and supplements may interact with Hepatitis A medications, and should be discussed with a healthcare provider before use.

Consult with a Registered Dietitian or Healthcare Provider

A registered dietitian or healthcare provider can provide personalized recommendations for maintaining proper nutrition and managing symptoms of Hepatitis A. Consult with a healthcare provider or registered dietitian to develop a personalized meal plan that meets your unique needs and goals.

Conclusion

Hepatitis A can be a challenging and complex illness, but with proper management and care, individuals can support liver function, manage symptoms, and promote overall recovery. This cookbook has been designed to provide individuals with Hepatitis A with a range of flavorful and nutrient-dense recipes, as well as meal planning and preparation tips to support proper nutrition.

However, it is important to remember that managing Hepatitis A requires a holistic approach that goes beyond nutrition. In addition to following a nutritious diet, individuals with Hepatitis A should focus on getting plenty of rest, staying hydrated, and avoiding substances that can further damage the liver. Regular exercise, stress reduction techniques, and close communication with healthcare providers can also be helpful in managing Hepatitis A and promoting overall health and wellbeing.

Furthermore, it is important to understand that Hepatitis A can have a significant impact on mental health and wellbeing. It can be challenging to cope with the physical and emotional symptoms of Hepatitis A, and individuals may feel isolated or overwhelmed during this time. It is important to seek out support from loved ones, mental health professionals, or support groups to help cope with these challenges and maintain a positive outlook.

In conclusion, managing Hepatitis A requires a comprehensive approach that prioritizes proper nutrition, rest, hydration, and mental health support. By following the recipes and meal planning tips in this cookbook, individuals with Hepatitis A can support liver function, manage symptoms, and promote overall recovery. With time, patience, and a holistic approach to care, individuals with Hepatitis A can regain their health and wellbeing

Made in United States
Troutdale, OR
01/09/2026